HIGH CHOLESTEROL
A Medical Fraud

INDO-VIETNAM
MEDICAL BOARD

Dr. Biswaroop Roy Chowdhury

Facebook: https://www.facebook.com/DrBiswaroopRoyChowdhury

YouTube channel: Dr. Biswaroop Roy Chowdhury

Website: www.biswaroop.com

Email: biswaroop@biswaroop.com

Edition: November 2018

Compilation:
Priyanka Agarwal

Graphics & Layout:
Shankar Singh Koranga

Brought to you by
Indo-Vietnam Medical Board
India Office:
C/o India Book of Records
B-121, 2nd Floor, Greenfields, Faridabad -121010
Ph. 01292510534, +91-9312286540
Vietnam Office:
C/o Bimemo
No 34/5 Tran Khanh Du Street,
Tan Dinh Ward, District 1, Ho Chi Minh City, Vietnam
- Hotline: (+84) 917540079 or (+84) 965947100
Malaysia Office:
C/o Bishwaroop International Healing & Research
Lot No. 2038 , Jalan Karak, 28500, Lachang,
Temerloh District Pahang Darul Makmur, West Malaysia
Tel : +60149056992
Switzerland Office:
C/o Nigel Kingsley
Kraftwerkstr. 95, ch-5465, Mellikon, Switzerland
Tel : 0041 79 222 2323

Published By:
Diamond Pocket Books
X-30, Okhla Industrial Area, Phase-II
New Delhi-110020
Ph.: 011-40712200
E-mail: sales@dpb.in Website: www.diamondbook.in

DEDICATION

Dedicated to my angel daughter Ivy,

loving wife Neerja

&

caring parents

Shri Bikash Roy Chowdhury

Shrimati Lila Roy Chowdhury.

CONTENTS

1

WHAT IS HIGH CHOLESTEROL!

If you already know it, then it will be easy for you to understand! However, if you are unaware about it, then it will be even easier!

As all that you know - is all wrong! Yes considerably wrong!

For your deep understanding, I have divided this topic into three parts,

Consensus...................The Argument!

Conspiracy..................The Strategem!

Cure...............................The Revival!

High Cholesterol

Consensus Conspiracy Cure

As I begin with the topic, in the meantime, you think over on two major questions!

1. Is Heart disease an infectious disease! Yes/No

2. Is High Cholesterol the causes of heart disease! Yes/No

Q.1) Heart Disease is an infectious disease

Q.2) High Cholesterol causes heart disease

What all be your answers to these questions, I am sure that they will certainly change by the end of your reading of this book!

Here to begin, let me introduce a short story of an egg!

Eggs as we all know when kept at 99^{0}F, 50%-60% humidity and proper environment; give rise to a new life. However, have you ever thought that, "what is the factor that creates a new life?"

A lab test can help you find out that 62% of the energy in an egg is cholesterol; actually it's the high level cholesterol!

However, if this cholesterol is lowered in an egg then no life can exist; therefore, it goes without saying that how essential cholesterol is!

Cholesterol is Life

Not only for the birth of a bird from an egg but even for us - humans!

Hence, for life to exist along with other molecules and chemicals; cholesterol is most crucial!

2

CONSENSUS

As we begin with this chapter, it is important to understand the various aspects of the cholesterol theory - from its discovery as a vital body molecule; to be a threat and disease causing agent, from the invention of statins - cholesterol lowering drug, to this becoming the most profitable drug in the world's pharmaceutical industry, there have been many phases of the cholesterol hypothesis.

When we say cholesterol to be a vital organic molecule, what does it signify? Even in pregnancy, it is very essential for the females to have high cholesterol to conceive and maintain a life within them! Therefore, it is cautionary for females not to intake any cholesterol lowering drugs during pregnancy.

For your knowledge, all the cholesterol lowering drugs have been categorized as "X-drugs," as given by the FDA, Food and Drug Administration. These are prohibited for females, as they may interfere with pregnancy and affect the development of fetus or incorporate deformities.

FDA
Statins are category 'X' drugs

The FDA being referred here is Food and Drug Administration, United States. It's not the FDA-India as they are mere followers of the FDA-United States.

Here, the most widely prescribed cholesterol lowering drug is Statins. You can conveniently find "statins" written over each pack of cholesterol lowering drug though under different brand names.

Astonishingly, the affects of cholesterol lowering drugs is no different on males; as it greatly increases the chances of in-fertility in men as well. These drugs increase the risk of Erectile Dysfunction by 51% in males, as given in the Journal of Clinical Pharmacy and Therapeutics, 1996. The chances of sperm abnormality rise by 11% in males, as given in the Reproductive Biology and Endocrinology, 2014.

Statins increase the risk of Erectile Dysfunction by 51 %

Journal of Clinical Pharmacy and Therapeutics' 1996 April 21

Statins increase sperm abnormality by 11 %

Reproductive Biology and Endocrinology 2014 July 2012

To sum up, as cholesterol is life and when being lowered, then it significantly impairs with the reproductive efficacy of both males and females. Even small consumption of this drug for some time can cause in-fertility, fetus deformities along with still births.

Adding to this, lowering of cholesterol has also been found to be associated with increased risk of breast cancer by 11 times in women, reported under Care Trial and published in the New England Journal of Medicine, 1996.

It should be notified that it's not 11%, but shockingly 11 times!

CARE TRIAL
11 times increased risk of a breast cancer **New England Journal of Medicine1996**

Also, it is crucial to mention that all the research work or trials being referred here are well established and approved by the FDA. These have a huge share in the management and regulation of the cholesterol lowering drugs.

You may find numerous journals and research studies worldwide with certain definite conclusions to support your theories. Yet again, every conclusion brings up contradictions! However, to get away with contradictions and arguments, I have only referred to those trials and research studies that are particularly approved by the FDA.

In this book, you will find the exact reference links of all the research studies and journals being referred by me. In a way, you can secure your understanding, build in a strong belief, confirm, affirm and spread the knowledge among others. As, it's common for doctors or medical associates to condemn this education; yet, with firm proof and understanding, you can become more convincing!

Here, sharing another evidence against the adverse affects of cholesterol lowering drugs. The FDA in 2012 issued a warning against the cholesterol lowering drugs, as they found 'Statins' to induce Diabetes, Muscle Damage and Memory Loss.

FDA Warning 2012
Statins may cause Diabetes, Muscle Damage and Memory loss

To understand the real meaning of may cause or 'induce', it becomes important to understand the medical language and its hidden implications. As, when they say the drug may cause certain side-effects, but, whether it will in your case or will not - is in itself an alarming question! Try to understand this trap, as it will surely adversely affect you, because in medical language using the word "definite" is prohibited. However, the reality that surrounds is that, "It will definitely have adverse affects on you!"

Appallingly, all the above side-effects or so diseases caused by cholesterol lowering drugs are life-threatening! However, if we talk about memory loss in particular, then it has its own attributes, as our brain is more than 50% of cholesterol! Not only this, the brain itself forms the cholesterol that it requires and to avoid wasting and sharing of this cholesterol formed by the brain into the body; there functions a Blood-Brain-Barrier.

Blood-Brain Barrier (BBB)

Astonishingly, though the brain is only 1% to 2% of total body weight, but its cholesterol utilization is 25% of that of the entire body.

To conclude, as you intake cholesterol lowering drugs; it affects the functioning of brain and leads to anxiety, memory loss and restlessness. It's important to mention that this is no hypothesis or a matter of chance but a definite occurrence. As by now, you all must have acknowledged that the brain mainly functions on cholesterol.

Now, this raises a question that if all the above evidences are apparently contradicting, then why are the cholesterol lowering drugs being widely prescribed by the medical associates!

The answer or plain reality rests in the Medical Culture. Yes, you read it right; it's not Medical Science that we depend upon, but the Medical Culture - a custom surrounding us. Like, 2×2 = 4. It is 4 in France, same in Germany or take any other country; this symmetry or system is called as Medical Science.

On the other hand, Medical Culture is a custom or tradition that varies from country to country and followed differently; like in India we follow Hindu Culture. These customs do not go after or depend on logics; as they themselves create logics or conventions. So, it's not Medical Science, it's simply a Medical Culture!

It's not Medical Science

It's a Medical Culture

For example, say if a person goes to a doctor with a condition of fatigue, so, here in India the doctor will suggest a blood sugar test. For the same condition in the US, a doctor will check the blood pressure, while in Germany the doctor will suspect a heart disease and conduct tests to diagnose cardiac-insufficiency. Again in Finland the doctor will chance upon cancer diagnosis and refer an oncologist, while a French practitioner will ask the patient to rest for a week and enjoy red wine!

Under medical practice, all the above approaches are correct and will relieve that person from his fatigue condition. However precisely, this is not Medical Science but Medical Culture! Again, culture doesn't lay a concrete pedestal; it requires no science, no logic, and no convention as a foundation. So, it is a mere name - Medical Science; whereas, in reality it's Medical Culture!

In a recent development I was fortunate to get associated with Dr. Smile from Smile Limited, Japan. Smile Limited is a big venture in Japan. In our conversations, I had to put forward a question conflicting my mind, which was as in India the death rate from heart attacks is the highest in the world, while the situation is just the opposite in Japan with lowest deaths from heart attacks. I asked over Dr. Smile for his opinion over such a variation.

His simple yet logical answer will leave you thinking! Much politely he replied that, in Japan to have a heart attack is perceived as you had a weak heart on the other hand to a have a brain stroke is perceived as you had a stronger sharper brain!

To understand this, firstly you must know that the death rates in a country are confirmed through death certificates that indicate or mention the cause or ailment behind the death of the deceased.

Even the World Health Organization, WHO refers to the death certificates to confirm the diseased-death rates in a country. Then, be it heart disease or brain strokes or any other ailment, WHO has no other means but to deduce their conclusions on the basis of available information on death certificates. But, is the provided information on death certificates completely reliable – is debatable!

Because in case of Japan, where heart attacks are listed lower than brain strokes, even though both heart attacks and brain strokes are caused by blockage of arteries, then how is it possible to have lowest heart attack rate and highest brain stroke rate in the same country?

In support of the above contradiction, a German Scientist proved that the information on death certificates with regards to the reason behind the death is 50% inaccurate, i.e., a general examination of the deceased cannot provide the real reasons behind the death. Only an autopsy can reveal the actual cause of death, which at an average is performed in 1 of 100 individuals in Japan. Whereas, it will be useless to comment over India with even limited number of Coroner's (the person who performs the autopsy).

About 1/2 of those whose cause of death was listed as 'Myocardial Infarction' in death certificate; died of something else.

Journal of American Medical Association-1979

Therefore, the estimations for diseased-death rates in a country on mere basis of information on death certificates is a critical submission. This helps me to conclude again that, this is not Medical Science, but Medical Culture, which inherits the influences of past, followed customs, traditions, rituals and laid beliefs!

Moving ahead to our prime topic, the basis of High Cholesterol!

Now, this started in between 1940s to 1950s, when the death rate from heart attacks was higher. A renowned nutritionist and scientist named Ancel Keys, was given the responsibility by the US government to find out the cause behind heart attacks. Moreover, the amount granted for the research was huge as approximately as 20,000 million dollars.

This took the scientist many years of hard work to collect data in support of his research. Finally in 1975, he presented his work through a graph plot of 7 major countries; this was referred as 7-Countries Study and reported that, "The population with lowest dependency on fats and cholesterol had lowest death probability by heart attack." In simple language, death rate is lower if the cholesterol is lower. Conversely, the population with high dependency on fats and cholesterol had higher death probability by heart attack!

Hence, for the first time, a new theory was accepted worldwide; high cholesterol or fat meant more diseases and low cholesterol or fat meant less diseases!

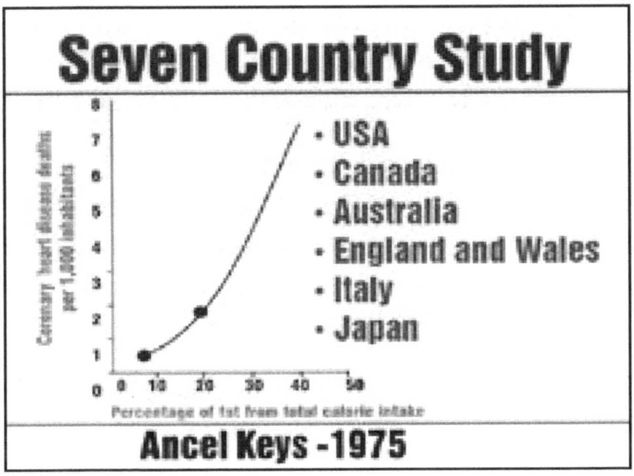

Let's assume the above report to be meaningful and begin with a new research. Let our research co-relate the number of deaths and the color of hair of the deceased people. For this study, we will try to find the number of deaths with grey hair! So, if we find that the maximum number of deaths had grey hair, then we shall conclude that grey hair cause death.

Subsequently, on the basis of our research and conclusion, we further present and recommend Black Dye to the masses, so as to retain black hair and reduce the chances of death!

Try to understand that, it is obvious that most deaths will have grey hair, hence they can be co-related. However, correlation cannot be the true cause; though may be a parallel cause but not the actual one!

Likewise, it's possible that the cholesterol is higher along with some heart disease like an aged person gets grey hair and possibly dies. So ironically, if we artificially color the person's hair black, then it will not decrease his age, so, how correlation is the cause!

Correlation
may not be the cause

Understand, medical science is based on assumptions, as for them, high cholesterol means high death rate, while low cholesterol means lower death rate, so, to lower the death rate lowering the cholesterol is a suitable goal.

Therefore, only on the basis of some odd correlation; all the cholesterol lowering drugs were approved. Subsequently, these drugs entered the market and were publicized among masses, keeping an account on observations and outcomes.

Like in our assumed theory, we marketed black dye, open for public use and observe its effects on death rate. The period of observation will be approximately 10 years, as followed in research studies. On the basis of the response throughout these years, we shall certain the required amendments. In the meantime, people, who are our resources for the experiment will keep on using black dye or 'cholesterol lowering drugs' and the positive or no-effect or in some cases even negative effects will continue. This is, what is Medical Science, though I call it as Medical Culture!

The trials for cholesterol lowering drugs were carried out in many countries that too for several years. The prime motto was to observe the difference between two groups. One of them was drug-dependent, while the other being drug-independent.

The major trials considered by the FDA were - LIPID 1998, WOSCOPS 1995, CARE 1996, Plac-1 & Plac-2 in 1995, Regress 1995, and KAPS 1995.

Thereafter, the meta-analysis of the data published in the New England Journal of Medicine 1998 concluded that, "Only one heart attack was prevented of every 172 individuals on cholesterol lowering drug-Statin for one long year."

Meta analysis of	
1)LIPID	**1998**
2) WOSCOPS	**1995**
3) CARE	**1996**
4) Plac -1	**1995**
5) Plac -2	**1995**
6) Regress	**1995**
7) KAPS	**1995**
New England Journal of Medicine 1998	

172 people taking Statin for 1 year will prevent only 1 heart attack

However, each drug-dependent individual had his own share of losses through the drug side-effects. In fact, at an average every drug-dependent individual will suffer from minimum two side-effects of the drug like bronchitis, anxiety, sleep-disorder, chest pain, cough, recurrent viral infections among other ailments. These symptoms further burden the health of the drug-dependent person and are left untreated by the doctors.

- **Edema**
- **Dermatitis**
- **Fatigue**
- **Chest pain**
- **Fever**
- **Weight gain**
- **Musculoskeletal Pain**
- **Muscle cramp**
- **Musculoskeletal Traumatism**
- **Dizziness**
- **Sleep disturbance**
- **Anxiety**
- **Pins and needles**
- **Urinary Tract Infection**
- **Upper Respiratory Tract Infections**
- **Cough**
- **Influenza**
- **Pulmonary Infection**
- **Sinus**
- **Bronchitis**
- **Blurred Vision**
- **Viral infection**

Besides, how can we certain that the one heart attack saved among the drug-dependent group was definitely due to the cholesterol lowering drug or for some other unevaluated reason. This in itself is a big question that goes without any answer or any research!

However, as we move further, there is yet another research that will definitely answer the above question.

The University of California and Los Angeles cumulated the data of heart attack deaths in 500 hospitals for approximately 20 years. The data included 1,36,905 heart attack deaths. Interestingly, they reported that of all the deaths, 75% patients had their cholesterol levels much below than the normal range. So, why the high cholesterol association with heart attacks theory of Ancel Keys did not have any similar findings. Where did the 7-Country Study reporting correlation between high cholesterol and death rate by heart attack came into picture!

Study by UCLA
75% of the patients hospitalized for heart attack had LDL Cholesterol less than 130mg/dl. American Heart Journal -2009
136905 patients

But, later on with more effective studies it was evident that heart attack had no correlation with high cholesterol levels!

The actual findings of Ancel Keys research were revealed in 1990's by a Deutsch Researcher, who reported the 7-Country Study to be in reality a 22-Country Study.

As you can see from the actual graph, there were 22 countries plotted for the analysis, wherein, Japan had the lowest heart attack death rate and lowest cholesterol levels, while USA had highest death rate and highest cholesterol levels. Whereas, in-between there were other countries at different positions plotted in the graph. See graph underneath.

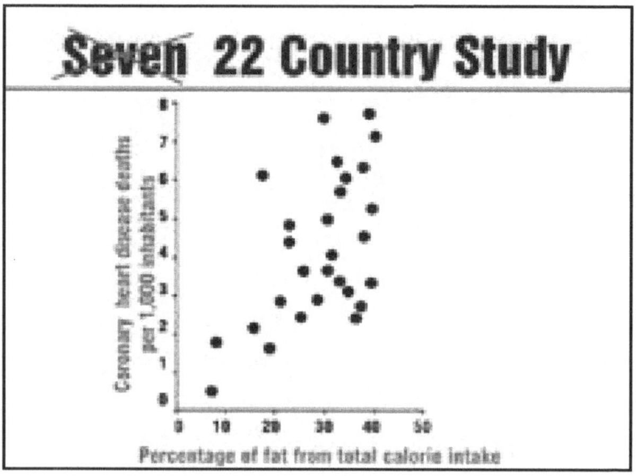

To a great extent, Ancel Keys tried so hard to present a correlation between high cholesterol levels and high death rate by heart attack that he only included those 7 countries that gave a linear plot on the graph and purposely ignored the remaining 15 countries as if they were insignificant. And, all this to only prove a convincing enough point that high is the cholesterol; higher be the death rate by heart attack.

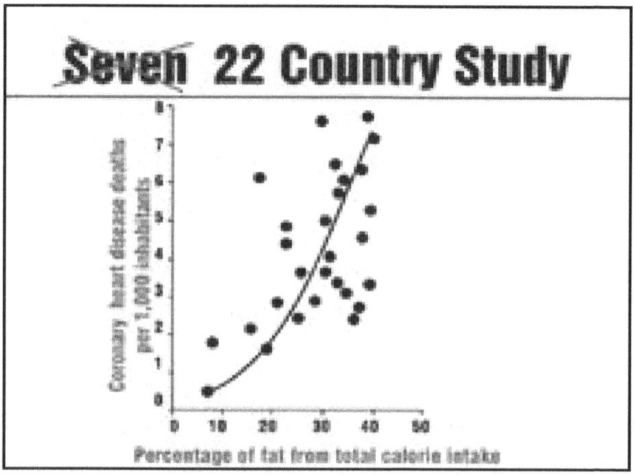

However, if a researcher had the choice and option to choose 7 other countries than those taken by Ancel Keys, then astonishingly, the graph plots just the opposite case, giving high cholesterol lowers the death rate by heart attack; this renders the research to be misleading and completely unreliable. Any research outcome must not support the researcher's or scientist's perception or convenience; they require firm foundation and must be in favour of the mankind.

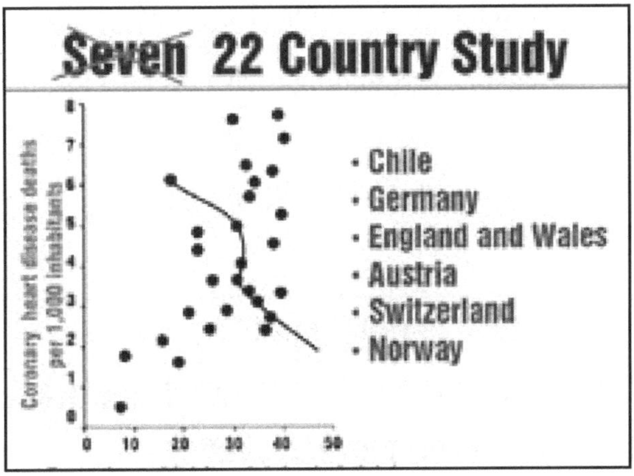

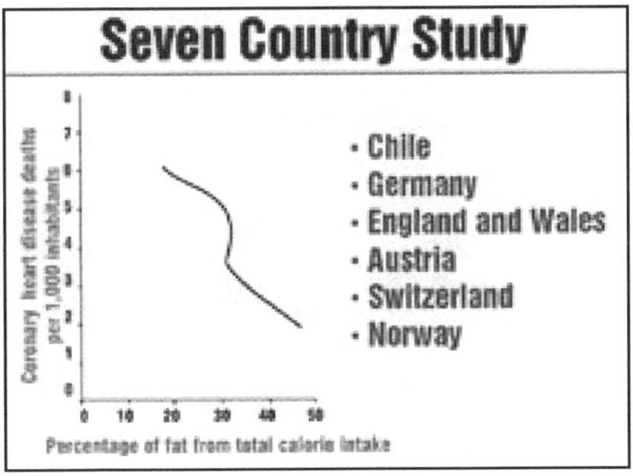

I am sure that by the above reference, you must be able to understand the basis that lay the high cholesterol menace! Unfortunately, by the time Ancel Keys actual research came into the limelight; the clutches of the cholesterol industry intensified.

With a firm understanding of the "Consensus or Agreement" about the introduction and regulation of cholesterol lowering drugs, next, we move on to the "Conspiracy" that surrounds the big question that, "Why even after so many compelling and undeniable evidences against the dangers of cholesterol lowering drugs, still they are widely prescribed and marketed by the medical agents!"

What was the reason surrounding such a support for this segment of drug and medical industry!

To understand this, we divide Conspiracy into two sections – Diagnosis and Drugs.

CONSPIRACY

Q1.) Why cholesterol lowering drugs are prescribed even more heavily ?

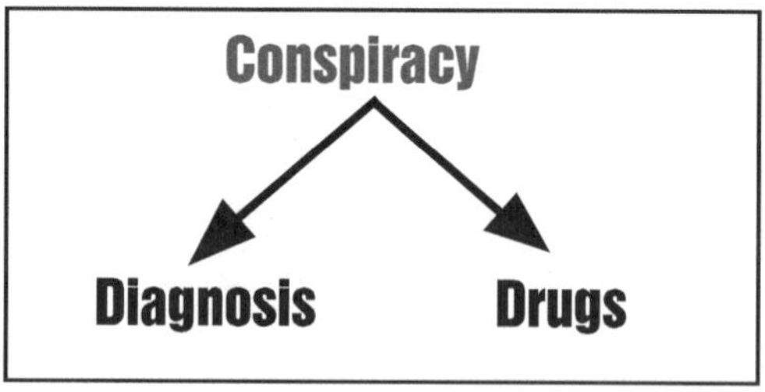

3

CONSPIRACY

Going back into the history of cholesterol diagnostic parameters, the body's optimum cholesterol value was accepted as ≤300mg/dl, as given by the Harrison Principle of International Medicine Edition VIII, 1977. The Harrison Principle of International Medicine is considered as the Bible of International Medicine which stated that, "Medical intervention may only be required when cholesterol levels exceeded 300mg/dl."

However, before 1988, in the European and US countries, there continued a dilemma with different thresholds for cholesterol levels (250mg/dl to 350mg/dl). In the year 1988, a 16 members committee named as Adult Treatment Panel 1 (ATP-1) was put forward by the US, to evaluate and decide the diagnostic parameters for cholesterol applicable to the entire population of the world. Subsequently, 240mg/dl was declared as the upper limit for cholesterol universally.

But, what is 240mg/dl of cholesterol level?

Let's assume my body has 5 liters of blood and my weight is 70 kilos. Then shall I require 5 bottles of 1 liter each to fill in the entire body's blood. If I take out 1 drop of blood from 1 bottle and check the cholesterol level, and if it comes out to be 200mg/dl, this means that 1 liter of my blood contains 2gms of cholesterol; the total cholesterol!

By the way how much is 2gms, 1 potato chip is 1gm, 2 potato chips is 2gms. So, if you get your cholesterol reading to be 200mg/dl, then this means that 1 liter of your blood has 2gms of cholesterol; the total cholesterol!

I hope that's clear, so, moving ahead, with 240mg/dl cholesterol limit, ATP-1 came up with another diagnostic parameter which was LDL, low density lipoprotein.

However, what do you understand by LDL, is it bad cholesterol or good cholesterol?

This is taken as bad cholesterol, as you all will agree!

Whereas scientifically, our body forms only the basic cholesterol; there are no variations like bad or good cholesterol. Let me explain this using an analogy of a person named Mr. Sharma, he is simply Mr. Sharma; not good Mr. Sharma or bad Mr. Sharma.

However, one day if he travels in an auto-rickshaw to office, gets late and looks very worn out and untidy; then we consider him as bad Mr. Sharma. While the same Mr. Sharma, when travels in a car to office, reaches on time and looks all gentleman, clean and in a 3-piece suit; then he becomes good Mr. Sharma.

Try to understand, this is entirely situational, the mode of transport and choice of clothing that he opts for makes him good Mr. Sharma or bad Mr. Sharma.

Similarly, the cholesterol formed by the body is the basic or the total cholesterol, but the mode of transport utilized by it to travel through the body makes it good or bad cholesterol. As, if it uses an auto to travel then it becomes the bad cholesterol, while if takes a car then it becomes good cholesterol.

The logic behind this theory is that, there isn't any good or bad cholesterol, it's only the total cholesterol formed by the body. While mode of transport is involved, however, it itself is controversial and thereafter tagging it to be good or bad is irrelevant.

If my subject, be it Mr. Sharma or the cholesterol travels by an auto, then it is even better as there will be less pollution, no parking problems and less investment. So, it depends on my perception of whether travelling by an auto or a car is beneficial.

Coming back to the introduction of LDL by ATP-1, with the introduction of LDL and 240mg/dl of cholesterol limit; 20% of world's population was now drug dependent in both the developed and developing countries (from 10% earlier).

Whereas in 1993, the Adult Treatment Panel 2 (ATP-2) apart from LDL and 240mg/dl of cholesterol limit, added the third diagnostic parameter termed as HDL or High Density Lipoprotein.

With total 3 diagnostic parameters given by ATP-1 and ATP-2, now the population dependent on cholesterol lowering drug or in the danger zone increased from 20% to 37%.

Time Line	**Total Cholesterol**	**% increase of Statin users**
Harrison Principle of International Medicine- 8th Edition, 1977	300	
Before 1988	250 - 350	10 %
ATP-1—1988	240+ LDL	20%
ATP-2– 1993	240+LDL + HDL	37%
ATP-3 – 2001	240 +LDL +HDL + triglycerides	48 %

This meant that each parameter affected double the population, especially above 40 years of age.

Yet again in 2001, ATP-3 introduced the fourth parameter, the triglycerides, and this along with LDL, HDL and the total acceptable cholesterol raised the population within the danger zone to be almost 48% of the total world's population.

Consequently, almost half or 50% of the total population especially above 40 years age of both the developed and developing countries were now high cholesterol patients.

This can be understood as, once my patient and now a diabetes educator, Mr. Vijay Yadav is a cricketer, a wicketkeeper, so, I challenged him to wicket me out.

With every ball, I kept on decreasing the height of the wickets and lastly removed the wicket itself; do you think this way had he ever been able to wicket me out, the answer is clear NO!

This was my scheme of action to avoid getting wicket out; the ATP cholesterol theory has the same plot.

As the present guidelines for cholesterol management recommend any and every person above 40 years of age to be medicated by cholesterol lowering drug, ruling out any requirement for examination for the LDL, HDL, triglycerides or total cholesterol levels.

This is the present criteria!

So, if you are 40 years above, then you can't be healthy and are labeled as diseased to be medicated by cholesterol lowering drugs for the rest of your life. This means that the wicket has been removed and there is no way to stump out!

Alas, the US based Adult Treatment Panel 1, 2 and 3 concentrated more on wealth than health of people, as you will further acknowledge.

Every year Fortune 500 presents the most profitable companies worldwide. After the establishment of ATP-3 model in 2001 and in the year 2002, Fortune 500 reported striking records. It showed that the 'top 10 Drug or Pharma companies had their profits even higher than the rest of the total 490 companies in records.'

Fortune Top 500 (2002)		
Top 10 Drug Companies' Profit	>	Top other 490 companies' profit
ATP-3 Impact		

The ATP-3 came out with huge profits for the drug and pharma companies building them stronger with big money!

The featured 10 drug companies were mostly US based, the origin grounds for Adult Treatment Panel. Merck, Johnson & Johnson, Pfizer, Bristol Myers Squibb, Pharmacia, Abbot Laboratories, Wyeth, Eli Lilly,

Top 10 Drug Companies	• Merck • Johnson & Johnson • Pfizer • Bristol Myers Squibb • Pharmacia • Abbot Laboratories • Wyeth • Eli Lilly • Schering-Plough • Amgen USA
ATP-3 Impact	

Schering-Plough, Amgen USA, these were the most profitable drug companies in 2002.

Not to finish, WHO in 2011 reported that, 60% of Heart, Cholesterol, Diabetes, Hypertension and Blood thinner medications are consumed by the Indians alone! Therefore, India's loss is the gain of top 10 pharmaceutical companies.

60% of CVD Drugs Consumed by Indians WHO -2011	• Merck • Johnson & Johnson • Pfizer • Bristol Myers Squibb • Pharmacia • Abbot Laboratories • Wyeth • Eli Lilly • Schering-Plough • Amgen USA
ATP-3 Impact	

Out of deep curiosity, I tried to find out those 30 members who constituted the ATP-3 association.

Of the total, 17 members were in connections with these 10 huge fortune drug companies. They were either posted as Scientists, Directors, Consultants or at other major designations. They being the agents and employees to the big name pharma companies also shared huge profits through these drug companies. So, the ATP mostly worked for the business development of pharma companies, therefore, how can we rely on their guidelines and blindly follow the ATP-3 model.

ATP -3 Panel Member profile

Member	Companies
Scott Grundy	Merck, Pfizer, Schering-Plough, Abbott Laboratories, Bristol Myers Squibb
Luther Clark	Abbott Laboratories, Bristol Myers Squibb, Merck, Pfizer
Margo Denke	Merck, Schering-Plough
Wm. James Howard	Pfizer, Merck, Schering-Plough, Abbott Laboratories
Donald Hunninghake	Bristol Myers Squibb, Merck, Schering-Plough, Pfizer
Roger Illingworth	Merck, Schering-Plough, Pfizer
Patrick Mc Bride	Pfizer, Merck, Abbott Laboratories, Bristol Myers Squibb
James Mc Kenny	Merck, Pfizer, Schering-Plough
Richard Pasternah	Merck, Pfizer
Neil Stone	Abbott Laboratories, Merck, Pfizer, Schering-Plough
Diane Becker	Pfizer
Linda Van Horn	Roche
Hollis Bryan Brewer	Merck, Pfizer, Schering-Plough
Steven Haffner	Pfizer, Merck
David Orloff	Bristol Myers Squibb, Merck, Pfizer, Wyeth, Abbott Laboratories, Eli Lilly

Member	Companies
Michael Proschan	Bristol Myers Squibb, Pfizer
J. Sanford Schwartz	Bristol Myers Squibb, Merck, Johnson & Johnson, Pfizer

Besides, we become the biggest sufferers of being dependent on these medications and drugs for several years. By this, not only our health but the nation as well suffers huge losses! Undoubtedly, these diagnostic guidelines and protocols are extremely disappointing.

Moving on to the drug discovery part, as to how the cholesterol lowering drug was introduced to the world!

The chief cholesterol lowering drug - Statin was invented by the scientist Endo in 1976. Before 1976, the cholesterol lowering drug was available in powder form; therefore its use was a little inconvenient.

In 1977, to further develop the medicine, scientist Endo partnered with two other scientists naming Goldstein and Brown. However, the partnership was soon over and surprisingly in 1980s, the same two scientists, Goldstein and Brown reported that "Statin causes Cancer."

1976 - Endo invented Statin (ML-236B)
1977- Endo Partnered with Goldstein and Brown to develop Statin
1980 - Brown & Goldstein publish paper that Statin causes Cancer

After the release of their research paper on "Statin causes Cancer", the cholesterol theory faced a set-back throughout the world, alongside; the Medical Industry had their mouths shut on promotions of Statins.

Nevertheless, it was the same time when the masses were deviated from the cholesterol theory to the introduction of heart by-pass surgery. During that time, heart by-pass surgery emerged as a fashion in the developed countries. This new medical technology was introduced as the only means to cure heart-diseases and patients were further burdened and drawn towards it in confusion and fear. With high treatment cost, this therapy was suitable for the moneyed and helped the Medical Industry to make good money from the by-pass surgeries.

Further on, in the year 1985, Goldstein and Brown were awarded with a Nobel Prize for 'Statins, a Cholesterol Lowering Drug.'

Baffled! Let me re-phrase. The same two scientists, who reported 'Statins to cause Cancer', were awarded with a Nobel Prize for their efforts and achievements in the development of the cholesterol lowering drug- Statin!

But, what about the research of 1980s for Statin's to show cancer causing characteristics, for what reasons the research and evidences were ignored and left out. Moreover, after 2 years in 1987, Merck Pharmaceuticals along with scientist Brown could get approval from FDA to manufacture Statins as cholesterol lowering drug.

1985 : Brown & Goldstein receive Nobel Prize for Statin related research but no mention of cancer.

1987 : Brown represents Merck in FDA to get approval of Statin.

Interestingly, in 2004, the first inventor of Statin, scientist Endo himself was found with a high cholesterol medical condition and surprisingly, he refused to use Statins for his own treatment, this was published in Wall Street Journal 2006.

2004: Endo himself did not use Statin to reduce his high cholesterol

Wall street Journal-2006

So, the biggest question of all times is that, "If the inventor himself denied the use of the drug for his own treatment, then why are you taking it?"

Yes, question yourself, why are you taking it!

Is it necessary or benefitting you by any means?

It is certainly worth throwing out, as no one in this whole world requires cholesterol lowering drugs.

With all the awareness of where this Statin originated or belonged to whom and what are its considerable affects; you can well understand that it's not at all needed!

While we're on the subject, there is a place in China where sun rays cannot reach and there is hardly any plantation. Some of the plants that survive adverse climate are eaten up by the insects or small animals of that place. But, there is one such small plant called as the 'Red Rice plant' which has special defensive abilities, as they defend themselves from insects by poisonous spray on them. It is even scientifically interesting, as to how some plants have such unique defense ability. The same features captured US Army's interest to be utilized for war and defense purposes.

When talking of war, you must know that Hitler was famous for his concentration camps. In his camps, mustard gas spray was used to decrease the immunity of people residing there, so as to deteriorate their health and thinking powers. This made the people almost lifeless, as their immunity and brain powers went to zero.

You will be surprised to know that the same transformed mustard gas is used in chemotherapy. Yes, this is no imagination or illusion because; if you don't believe my words, then refer to the medical journals, where you will get all the reports and evidences supporting the same.

Anyhow, at least now you can entitle Hitler to be real the inventor of chemotherapy (mockingly)!

Getting back to the Red Rice plant's defense ability, so as to find out whether its poison can be used against prisoners and warriors, the US Army began to research, and the results were alarming! As, the poison was reported to be Statin and it was confirmed that, with small dosages to humans will lead to slow death, infertility, memory loss, cancer, an endless list of life-threatening diseases.

This is the same Statin taken by all of you!

Still, will you believe in Medical Science, while in reality it is Medical Culture!

It's a culture driven for the profits of some people, alike superstitions, that are morally destructive than constructive. Similarly, some rules and values are only practiced for the benefits of one segment of people, not for the mankind. Moreover, we being mere followers are the plain victims, who are misguided with relation to logics, theories and most importantly fear!

Even in India, it's a crime to support that, "Diabetes or High Cholesterol (you may need to lower cholesterol if it is >300mg/dl) or Hypertension can be cured without medications and medical treatments."

Yes, it's a harsh reality! If you try to go against it and reveal its real picture, then this well rooted system can send you behind the bars. Even they tried to detain me thrice! Moreover, some of our diabetes educators have even been arrested and released. Alongside, I come across many legal notices against my work to threaten and suppress me and my mission, because, as you challenge the medical industry and offer a better cure with disease-free life, then they will definitely try to oppose you and thrash you!

Even in the history of our culture, whenever a reform or a superstition was challenged by a group of people like us, then they had to face oppositions and difficult situations, but, somebody has to initiate the change, be it you or me!

Often I see people rejecting my seminar passes only by reading 'Cure without Medicines.' According to them, this is impossible. Sadly, they have been trained to depend on medications from long and perhaps have become comfortable within this trap. As we as humans are more emotional than intellectual, and are comfortable with the common customs and trends being constantly followed!

However, let me remind you that our medical industry's model is similar to our customs and religion. So, ironically, we follow a Medical Religion, which is certainly no good for any of us!

Therefore, we must accept the reality and try to free ourselves from the clutches of this conspired medical religion. To begin so, the important question is, "What shall be done to lead a disease-free life?"

4

CURE

To start with 'Cure', let's understand some fundamental concepts with a new approach for better understanding.

At this point, it's clear that our prime aim is to prevent heart diseases as well as, look for the complete cure. Therefore, in this chapter along with steps to 'Cure', you will also find some more significant references. Though I understand that my theories may seem to be completely contradictory to what you have been taught, learnt or told about. However, you may come up with arguments and research more on the matter to finally understand, believe and propagate in this direction. Apart from that, I am all open for your questions and any discussion.

Women's health around the world has always been a matter of concern. The British Medical Journal 2007 proclaimed as the most authentic journal reported that, "There is no impact of cholesterol on death rate by heart disease in women." This study was the meta-analysis of 19 different research work that involved 1,24,814 women and concluded that, "There is no connection between cholesterol and heart disease on women's health."

Meta-analysis of 19 study (124814 women) cholesterol had no impact on heart disease or death

British Medical Journal –2007, May 12

For instance, there is no connection between shoe size and heart disease. But, if we say that those with a smaller shoe size won't suffer heart disease and those with bigger size will have heart complications and thereafter, insanely invent a novel shoe to forcefully reduce the shoe size!

Like our shoe sizes are variable and have no connection with heart disease, similarly, there exists no connection between cholesterol and heart disease in women.

The National Heart, Lung and Blood Institute established by the US Government is in sync with the same theory and after analyzing 80,000 women reported that, "There was no impact of cholesterol levels on women's health." Therefore, through scientific studies it's evident that women need not worry or concern about their cholesterol levels, and I am sure that, "50% of women patients will become non-patients by mere acknowledging these studies!"

NHLBI
Study on 80,000 women **No impact on women** **Circulation 1992**

The above theory is no different for men; as similar studies have stated that, "Even at above 50 years of age, there is no impact of cholesterol levels on heart functions." There is indeed a slight reference with regards to high cholesterol and heart disease in men below 50 years of age, however, that doesn't indicate that lowering this raised cholesterol through medication is any beneficial. As for men below 50 years of age, to reduce the cholesterol levels through medical intervention is proven to be even more harmful. It causes the same effect as we dye/color our hair black and assume that we are getting younger.

From the Clofibrate, British Heart Journal 1978 to the latest the Evacetrapib Accelerate trial 2016, along with many other trials confirmed the same theory that, "The cholesterol lowering drugs only lower the cholesterol readings but not the associated diseases."

Cholesterol lowering drugs trial		
1st	1978	Clofibrate British Heart Journal
Last	2016	Evacetrapib ACCELERATE

As to lower the readings (the number value) and expect it to reduce the possibility of associated diseases and risk factors are two different aspects.

Like, there is a Biofeedback Tester for Happiness that shows the current state of mind of an individual. When tested in-between fingers, it detects the electrical signals from the body and converts them in digital readable form. High readings denoted depressed state of mind, low readings – happiest state or else normal to high anxiety states.

Now, a tube or cream is introduced for the depressed people with high readings, with a conception that, when applied before the test it will change the depressed state to happy state with low readings. Thereafter, depressed people start using it, applying it in-between fingers and testing; and whoa, it shows desirable results.

What a magical cream with significant effects, changes depressed state to happy state (high readings to low readings). What an invention, a blessing by science!

But, you may never know the reality or trick that surrounds the introduction, application and effects of the above said cream.

When the miracle cream is applied before taking the test, it acts as a barrier and minimizes the transfer of electrical signals from the body to the tester. Thereby, the device shows lower readings owning to happy state of mind. While your state remains the same, but readings are definitely low. In this case, a person may never know the hidden business of the cream and will use the cream forever, assuming it to be the reason for his happiness.

This is a clear case of playing with the psychology of patients and is termed as a business of fear, or disease mongering.

Disease mongering is not uncommon and started in the year 1985 by Dr. Joseph Lister. He was a surgeon by qualification and owner to cement and floor cleaner manufacturing units. During the times of business lows, Dr. Lister started marketing the floor cleaner solution into small bottles as mouth cleaner.

Initially the plan did not work but for the next 5 years, he promoted the disease called 'Halitosis' which is 'bad breath' and simultaneously his product gained recognition. The product is still in the market by the name of 'Listerine' and many of you must be regular users of it.

Unfortunately, in disease mongering, a disease is being created and unnecessarily hyped for the profits of a particular group of people. Moreover, it's further promoted by spreading fear among people for that particular disease.

High Cholesterol is also a disease mongering case!

As explained earlier, among males below 50 years of age, high cholesterol may indicate slight risk of heart disease, but to reduce this cholesterol with statins to reduce the risk of heart disease is a misconception!

Yes, this is a false belief!

Nonetheless, they want you to keep on taking statins, so the business keeps on flourishing!

But, what is the way out?

How to protect the heart otherwise!

A protection to an extent that within a week's time, you will be forced to throw away your blood pressure, cholesterol and blood thinners pills!

Step 1 : Throw away the 'Statins'.

With Step 1, you have to throw away and get rid of Statins completely; you don't need them.

Step -1
Throw the STATIN

But first, it's important to understand the action mechanism of statins, how statins actually work inside the body.

When we breathe in oxygen and throw out carbon dioxide, this CO_2, in presence of sunlight and water is utilized by the plants to get glucose. Glucose is the major nutrition. In our body, as we consume a plant food in form of fruits or vegetables, this glucose gives rise to a series of chemical reactions within the cell leading to the formation of many crucial metabolites. One of this important metabolite is cholesterol, as you can understand from the picture below –

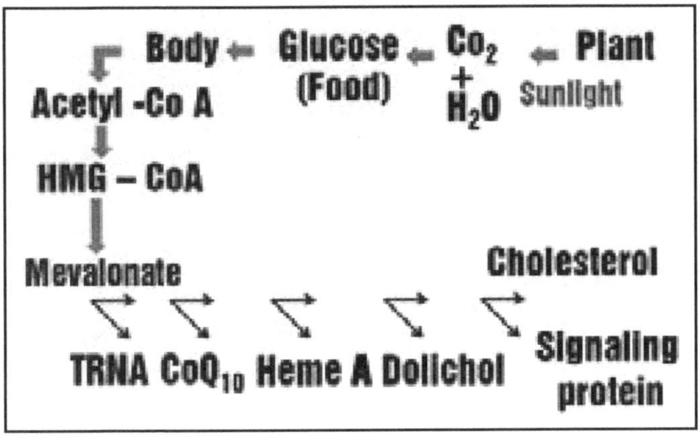

When on statins, the drug acts by blocking the metabolic pathway at such a point that apart from cholesterol, many important reactants and products are not synthesized.

One of the very crucial metabolite is CoQ10, which works as a spark plug for the heart, without which the heart function is impaired and gets weakened.

Another is tRNA, lack of this metabolite leads to development of cancer in the body.

Yet another is the signaling protein, which is essential for appropriate working of the entire signaling system to function as per the stimuli.

To further explain, when you feel hungry and take an apple in your hand, the brain starts sending signals to the organs for food digestion.

In case of pancreas, it is signaled to produce insulin, but if the signaling protein's production is less, thereby the complete signaling system will be weak and in case of pancreas, it may not secrete the required amount of insulin, only leading to high sugar in the blood, which is then diabetes!

Such is the importance of each and every metabolite through every metabolic pathway.

To understand better, take an example of a red rose with many leaves and thorns. Is it possible to only cut the thorns, keeping the leaves safe? Practically Not!

As hard as you try, you will end up cutting the entire stem!

Similarly, in order to cut or block the cholesterol, many other crucial derivatives also get blocked from the pathway.

And the scissor here is the cholesterol lowering drug, Statin.

Sadly, we are never told about these concepts, that by taking statins:-

1. The cholesterol will be lowered, whether it will benefit you or not.
2. And, the entire pathway will be affected losing its vital metabolites for body processes.

The scientific name for Statins is HMG CoA Inhibitor, not the cholesterol inhibitor, so the name itself signifies the difference in its action mechanism. As it acts upon the HMG CoA substrate and not just the body's cholesterol!

It may shock you that in children whose bodies do not synthesize this chain suffer from a rare disease known as Hutchinson-Gilford Progeria Syndrome (HGPS), which leads to premature aging in children as much as eight times faster than normal with a shorter lifespan (remember the movie 'Paa'. Thus, it can be foreseen that this critical pathway will have same aging affects on us as well.

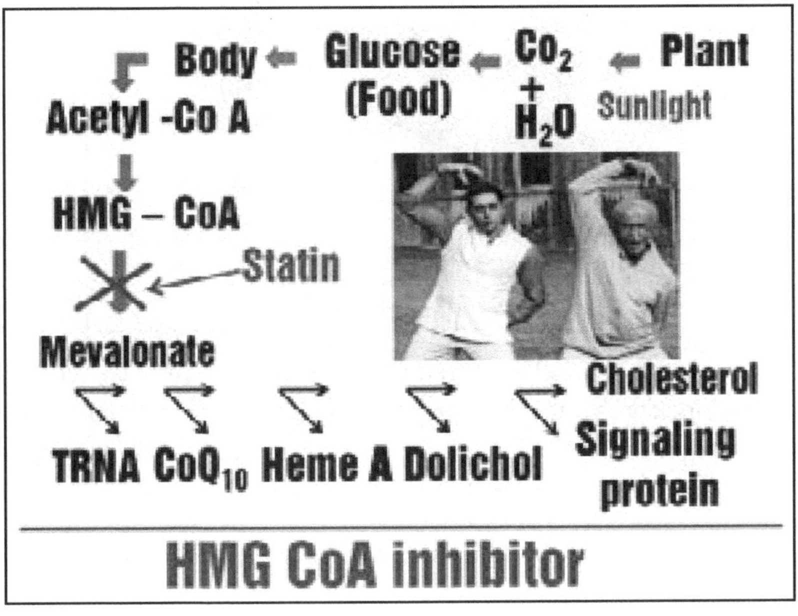

Coming back to heart and cholesterol, so, why do we get heart diseases?

According to medical science, it is due to the deposition of cholesterol in the arteries causing blockages.

Now, assume that a building gets demolished in front of you; and all you can see now is the bricks as debris. However, bricks are the building blocks of the building and cannot be suspected as the cause behind the pull down of the building. Same is with cholesterol, because if high cholesterol leads to heart disease; then people with low cholesterol should never have a heart condition, which is totally the opposite case, as low cholesterol people have more heart diseases.

So, how is only cholesterol suspected for artery blockages?

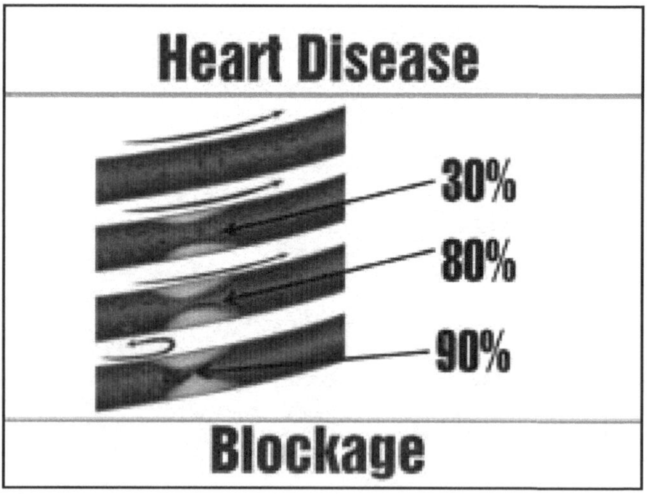

Other way, it is also questionable that why aren't the veins getting blockages but only arteries do, though both have cholesterol circulating through the blood.

For your understanding, arteries carry blood from the heart to other organs of the body and veins carry blood back to the heart from the body's other organs.

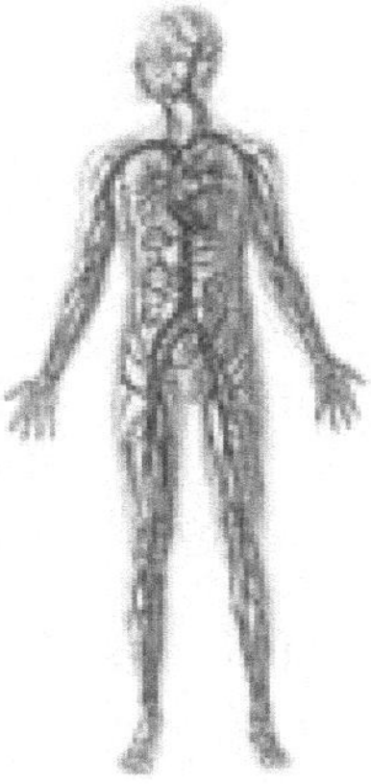

Why no blockages in veins

But again, what actually causes heart diseases?

What causes heart disease?

This brings me to share with you 3 major clues to understand the heart disease concept well:-

- First, Circulation 2006, concluded to have found 50 different bacterial species at the site of heart blockages.

Clue-1
50 different bacterial species are found in blockages **Circulation 2006**

- Second, the American Journal of Cardiology 2002 stated that, the temperature of blockages is higher than normal body's (arteries) temperature. This is a case when we have elevated body temperatures during an infection; this is the body's defense mechanism against the foreign invaders or to counter the infection.

Clue-2
The Temperature of blockage is higher **American Journal of Cardiology 2002**

- Thirdly, the New England Journal of Medicine 2004 concluded that, 1/3rd of heart attack patients had some infectious disease before the heart attack.

Clue-3
1/3 of the Heart Attack patients had infectious disease immediately before heart attack **New England Journal of medicines 2004**

More or less, the above 3 declarations have enough answers to explain the causes behind heart diseases.

However, these evidences were not available before the year 2000, it was only after this year that the medical science could get the supporting data.

To understand the factors that contribute and prevent the heart diseases, we must first analyze all the above 3 reports and comprehend their conclusions.

Our bloodstream along with other constituents also circulates germs that keep on attacking the endothelial layer of the blood vessels. Endothelial is the inner most layer of the blood vessels and keeps in constant contact with the blood and its constituents, even cholesterol.

The strength of this endothelial wall depends on optimal production of Nitric Oxide (NO) in the body as it is one of the most vital molecules with key roles especially in cardiovascular health.

But, if NO production remains low in the body then it leads to weakening of the endothelial wall which is termed as Endothelial Dysfunction.

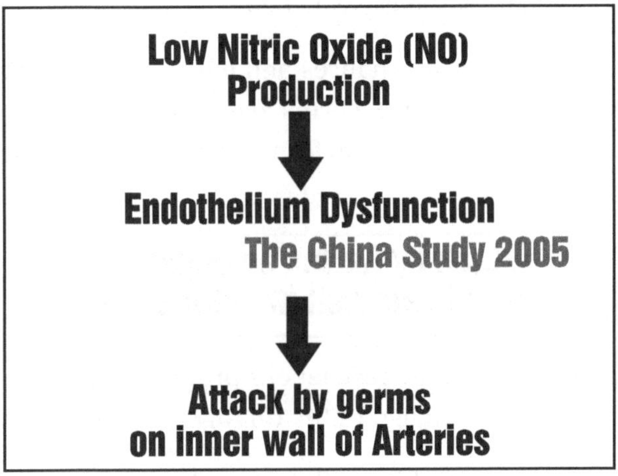

Alongside, in our body, the blood pressure in arteries is 100 times more than the blood pressure in veins. In other words, the pressure inside the walls of the arteries is 100 times higher than the pressure

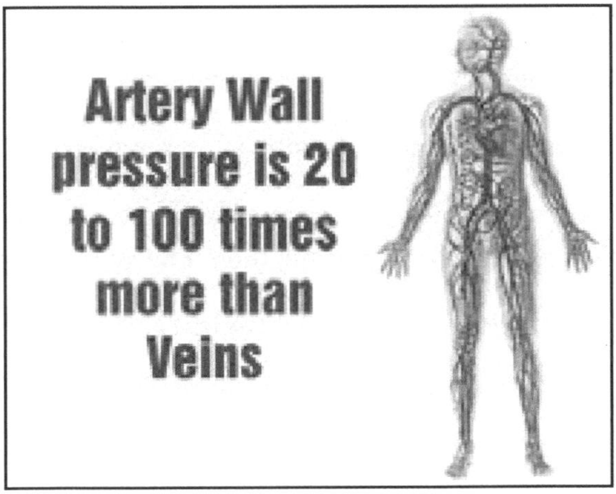

at the walls of veins. It's like a balloon filled with air, if we increase the air pressure inside, then equal pressure will be exerted on the inner walls of the balloon.

So, the condition is:-

1. Pressure is high

2. Endothelial layer has weakened

This leads to increased chances and effects of germ attack in the blood vessels. In such a case, germs keep on attacking, accelerating the rate of damage which leads to formation of wound at the damaged site.

Attack by Germs on weak arteries/inner wall inflammation

At the site of the wound, a rescuer or a protective agent accumulates to heal and mend the damaged site - this agent is Cholesterol!

The role of cholesterol is to always protect the heart and not to cause any damage to the heart.

But then how do we get blockages!!

The series of events are such –

1. Constant germ attack

2. Accelerated damage at the site

3. The rescuer cholesterol accumulates to heal the site, but if this goes on for a long period of time; then it becomes a blockage!!

This simple attack and rescue mechanism going on in the arteries leads to blockages, giving way to heart disease or heart attack.

To sum up, it is attack by germs on weak arteries causing inner wall inflammation. It is infection wining over cholesterol giving way to formation of blockages. It is important to note that inflammation in itself is not a disease; it is simply a repair and rescue mechanism of the body.

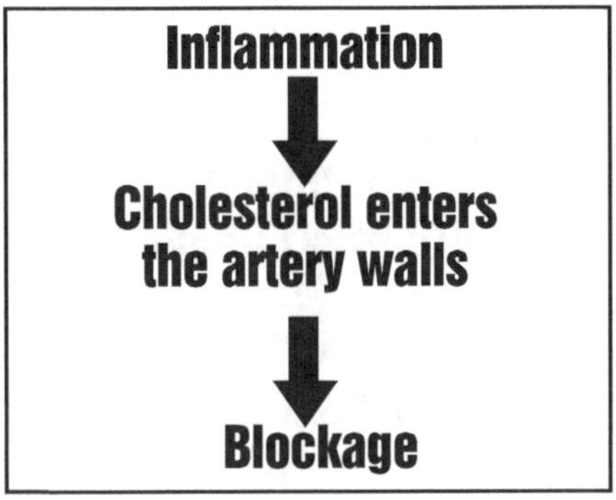

By now you must have understood that all these events of germ attack, inflammation, cholesterol accumulation and following, started with one major cause i.e. the weakening of the endothelial wall. But, what causes endothelial wall to weaken? The weakening of endothelial wall is due to low nitric oxide production in the body. So, whenever the nitric oxide production is low, but the blood pressure in arteries remains high, then the attack by germs is amplified leading to the formation of wound at the particular site.

Now, we know the real cause behind the heart diseases and blockages, which is not cholesterol but a condition lead by different factors. However, now to look for the solution, which is definitely not the cholesterol lowering drug - Statin.

So, what's the solution?

It is simply "Nitric Oxide" (NO)

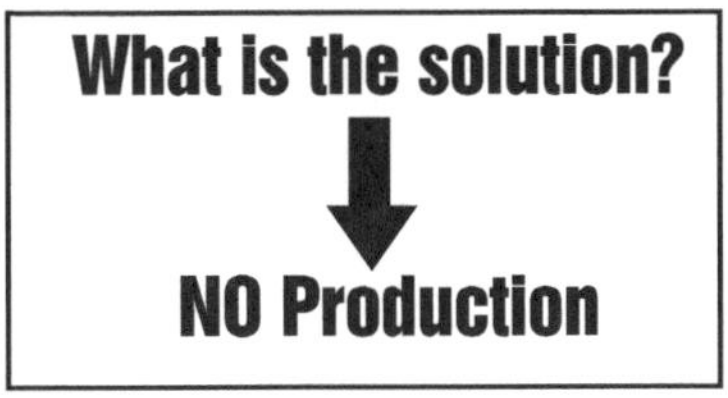

By only increasing the nitric oxide production; all the factors can be balanced. With this, I want to give you a miracle formula - "Formula to cure Heart Disease." This will equip you to enhance nitric oxide production in the body to protect your heart.

Formula to
Cure Heart Disease

↓

Increased production
of NO

Step 1:- As was given earlier to throw away the "Statins."

This is because along with other damaging effects, statins also restrict nitric oxide production. Many a times, patients have this concern, "Can I continue with statins and start over the diet!"

It is crucial to stop statins, as they interfere with nitric oxide production, thereby putting you back to point zero!

Step 2- Increase the production of Nitric Oxide.

But, how to do this, simply by making food the major source of nutrition!

- Start with Fruit Breakfast

Quantity: Weight ×10gms of fruit breakfast till 12 noon.

For example, a 70kgs person must consume 70×10gms = 700gms of any 3-4 variety of fruits that are readily available in the market.

Formula to cure Heart Disease
Breakfast : **weight in kg X10=___gms** **of fruits in breakfast**
Step-2

Also, there is no restriction on choice of fruit; seasonal fruits are relishing and fit well to pocket, or it can be any fruit that suits your taste. There are no restrictions for diabetic patients as well; they may enjoy mangoes and sugarcane juice without any fear because this fruit breakfast will not raise the blood glucose levels rather will normalize it without any adverse effects. Many of our diabetic educators were previously diabetic and now are completely cured and eat and enjoy great well-being. During our diabetes reversal tours, participants follow the same diet instructions and gradually results are apparent; giving them a diabetes free life!

The fruits can be taken in small quantities throughout (you may start anytime after waking up) till 12 noon. Only the weight is important, so measure the consumable quantity after peeling or removing seed(s) if any - this should be your weight into 10 grams.

For instance, my work involves extensive travelling and staying out, so, to manage the diet routine, I religiously carry a dozen of bananas in my bag and mostly look for fruits and vegetables easily available in that country or place. The point is that, this diet can be followed with any work routine, anywhere, anyplace.

However, make sure your breakfast contains 'no' chapatti, curd, vegetables, bread, tea or any other eatable; it must only comprise of complete fruit indulgence.

- For Lunch & Dinner, you have to get ready with 2-plates.

Plate 1: This must consist of 3-4 varieties of raw vegetables – carrot, peas, tomatoes, cucumber, capsicum, bell peppers etc.; you may create a list of your own. It may also include par-boiled vegetables like broccoli, cauliflower, potatoes or beans along with some raw green leafy vegetables like spinach, coriander or lettuce.

Quantity: Weight ×5gms = Plate 1

Formula to cure Heart Disease
Plate -1 Lunch/Dinner weight in kg x 5= __gms of vegetables
Step-2

Plate 2: This is the 'my wish plate' as you may add anything of your taste – be it dosa, idli, chappati, cooked vegetables/beans/pulses or even junk food as a treat.

Quantity: No limit!!

Instructions: First to consume entire Plate 1; then as per the appetite go for the Plate 2.

Note: Plate 1 is indispensable and cannot be avoided, you have to consume Plate 1 completely; thereafter you can indulge in Plate 2.

Plate 2 is to be taken as 'filler' for leftover hunger; this plate is completely avoidable and must be dropped if not required.

One may think that after consuming high quantity of raw vegetables, there will hardly be any urge to eat Plate 2. Bingo!! This is the only idea behind, that there remains no requirement or hunger for Plate 2.

You may find this routine difficult for 2-3 days in the beginning, but post that, your body will start to crave more and more of this kind of diet; because the diet is more water so it makes you feel light and eat more often.

Your weight especially belly fat or rigid body fat will reduce drastically during the course of this diet. For those with balanced health may start over with a little less quantity, say if by weight you require 350gms, then you may begin with 300gms of raw intake in lunch and dinner exclusively.

However, by any chance, Plate 2 cannot be taken before Plate 1. By this your outcomes will be no better rather can be worse!

Only after consumption of Plate 1, Plate 2 can be started; this system is the same for lunch and dinner.

Step 3 : Stop consuming cholesterol food.

You have to get away from food that provides cholesterol to the body. This step is highly significant because it's crucial to distinguish between food with cholesterol and food without cholesterol.

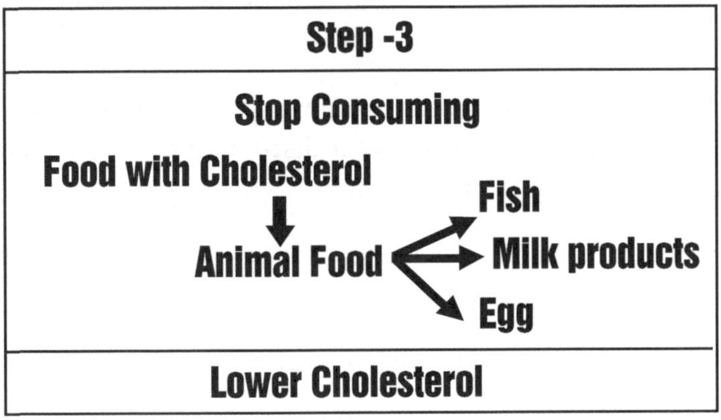

It is to understand that among plants and animals, only animals can form cholesterol, whereas, plants and their products are devoid of cholesterol. Therefore, by following the construction of nature to get rid of cholesterol food; one must stop consuming animal food and products.

We have been brought up with the belief that cow's milk is healthy, it's correct; it is healthy; but for the calf, for you it's a source of cholesterol and needs to be eliminated from the diet.

Try to understand, humans are the only animals that intake milk throughout their lives and for that depend on other animal's milk. None of the other animal uses other animal's milk neither do they require throughout their lives.

So, spare yourself from depending on other animal's milk; rather milk consumption is not required at all, it is only essential for the new born to be on mother's milk for 2 years.

Nature has directed us this way, so we depend on mother's feed for nutrition for initial years. That's all. To depend on milk for life throughout as core nutritional intake is just a fake perception/build-up/myth. Hence, with step 3, you have to get yourself completely rid of any kind of animal product, milk and its products as well.

Once you start to apply step 3; automatically, your cholesterol will get balanced.

You can now stop rather throw away your cholesterol lowering pills. If in case, your family or doctor discourages you from stopping the pills, ask them one simple question!

Ask them, of who takes the responsibility of your health, whether it's your family or your doctor?

Ask them if I continue the pill, then who assures me safe health or in other case if I discontinue with the pills, then who will stand for my health!

In both the cases, neither your doctor nor your family is responsible for your health and well being.

You may find a good percentage of population dying from heart attack even after being on cholesterol lowering pills. Who is responsible or will take charge for this, a doctor will never!

A doctor simply prescribes a pill, knowing the side effects all well. He will not discuss or encourage you to take the track of healthy eating and good lifestyle because it is convenient to write a prescription note letting an individual to be dependent on medicine for the rest of his life, than to take charge!

It is definitely difficult, and no doctor will guide you to implement the natural cure or discourage the use of pills.

Your health is your responsibility, no doctor, no pill will guarantee you a good safe health, be on a pill or not!

Whereas, this diet treatment gives you complete guarantee; it keeps you away from the lethal effects of drug along with drug side-effects. The best cure is within, as you connect more with the truths of nature and life-style; you will lead your life and health more responsibly.

Take the responsibility now, understand, comprehend and bring the change for your good-self.

5

CONCLUSION

All the facts and figures given throughout the book are backed up by scientific research. One can easily access multiple medical forums to conclude the myths about cholesterol theory and get firm with the given solutions.

To make your belief more concrete, here are some more examples.

A major research, the OSLO Study of 1975 conducted for several years and published in Acta Medica Scandinavica reported that, “In a population, healthy cholesterol levels can be maintained by complete elimination of animal food from the diet.”

Interestingly, the study also reported that, “In a population with healthy cholesterol levels, the death rate by heart attack remains unaffected.” This meant that body’s cholesterol level had no association with the death rate by heart attack, thereby showing no correlation.

OSLO -1 Study
Year - 1975 Publication: Acta Medica Scandinavica

On the same grounds, the OSLO Study 2 of 2006, published in The Journal of Norwegian Medical Association reported that, “In a population, both the cholesterol level and the death rate by heart attack can be lowered by complete elimination of oil and animal food especially milk from the diet."

OSLO - 2 Study
Year - 2006 **Publication:** **The Journal of Norwegian Medical Association**

This point is crucial, as for the protection of heart and balancing the cholesterol; oil intake must be lowered.

Because, Less Oil = Reduced chances of Heart Disease.

The plant-based diet therapy given in Step 1, 2 and 3 is in line with the OSLO Study, where till 12 noon with fruits, the oil intake is zero, while lunch and dinner comprise majority of raw vegetables minimizing the oil consumption through Plate 2.

The importance of diet therapy has been illustrated by many major research studies, of them the recent and well recognized is the Lyon Diet Heart Study published in the Archives of Internal Medicine. This trial was conducted from 1995 to 2005 with 2,14,284 men and 1,60,012 women subjects in Lyon, France.

Lyon Diet Heart Study
214284 Men **160012 Women** **Time :1995 - 2005** **Place: Lyon, France** **Archives of Internal Medicine**

According to this study, in a population with dietary modifications following results were obtained:

23% reduction in death...

21% reduction in cancer...

24% reduction in heart disease...

Therefore, you can now easily relate to the strength of the diet treatment.

This plant-based diet is highly impactful and comes with a warning for drastic improvements. A timeline of expected outcomes once you start over with the diet therapy are briefed as under:

Timeline	
24hrs to 72hrs	Diabetes
3 days to 1 week	High Blood Pressure, High Cholesterol, Intestinal disorder
1 month	Obesity, Heart Diseases
2 month	Thyroid Disease
6 month	Cancer, Asthma, Arthritis
8 month	Skin Disorder, Kidney dysfunction, Liver disorder

In first 24 to 72 hours, the blood glucose levels will normalize and you will be forced to stop the blood sugar medicines and insulin if prescribed.

In 3 days to one week, high cholesterol, high blood pressure will normalize along with relieving intestinal disorders. You will be forced to discontinue your medicines otherwise it will lead to conditions like extreme low blood pressure. As, with the plant-based diet, the patients are compelled to give away their medicines to avoid low sugar and/or low blood pressure, which are even more fatal.

In first one month, drastic symptomatic relief is observed with heart ailments. A feeling of strength in heart and body makes a person walk, jog, climb stairs, control breathing and exercise without fear. Obesity, the most prevalent medical condition becomes history in one month of the diet therapy; patients also experience a sense of balance in the body with motivated and peaceful mind, leading to faster recovery.

In first two months, thyroid subsides and once a TSH test indicates normal thyroid levels, thereafter, you can cut down or stop away with your thyroid medicines completely.

In first six months, complicated respiratory illnesses like asthma and major allergies of several years settle down, giving a new life to lungs with complete detoxification and restoration.

These six months can get cancer patients a new life, as even advanced stage cancer surrenders with the effect of plant-based diet treatment. Within the same time frame, arthritis and associated discomforts subside.

In first eight months, improvements and complete revival are observed with skin disorders, kidney dysfunction and liver disorders.

The above results are not imaginary, but, have been experienced by our Diabetes Educators', who are well trained and have good experience with plant-based diet therapy and diseases. Their experiences with their patients have been presented in the book 'Diabetes Educators' Success Stories, wherein, you can learn the real experiences of our Diabetes Educators' on diseases and cure with their patients. Nevertheless, the book also contains feedback of patients with prescription details on disease(s), their history, symptoms and present conditions along with their personal details which you may use to contact them and get more affirmed and confident on how their diseases moved towards healing. This unique collection of real stories through the patients and diabetes educators' will remove all your dilemmas and will certainly give you a kick start on plant-based diet treatment.

These patients suffered from cancer, heart diseases, thyroid, blood pressure, cholesterol, asthma and allergies, obesity and majorly diabetes. Why majorly diabetes, because with diabetes itself other conditions like obesity, thyroid, high cholesterol, blood pressure and organ dysfunction are commonly associated, therefore, the body experiences a combination of disturbances.

After elaborating the scientific and practical aspects of plant-based diet and with a hope that now you must be ready for a new beginning towards healthy being, here it becomes important to understand that as to how far any medical invention is necessary.

Are medicines really required or do they really help?

To this, 4 major trials are referred and listed, these are - Diabetes Prevention Program - DPP for Pre-diabetes in 2002, Accord for diabetes in 2008, ALLHAT for blood pressure in 2002 and IDEAL for kidney in 2010.

Year	Trial	Disease
2002	DPP	Prediabetes
2008	ACCORD	Diabetes
2002	ALLHAT	B.P.
2010	IDEAL	Kidney

The ACCORD trial had 10,000 participants and was funded by governments of US, Canada and U.K. The trial clearly reported that, "High blood sugar is bad, but to keep it low with medicines is worst."

Also, much stress was given to the importance of symptomatic diagnosis to decide on the requirement of medical intervention.

Exemplifying, one of my diabetic patients Mr. S. K. Gupta drove to my clinic and back in his car with a sugar as high as 586! Commonly, this range of sugar will show many dangerous symptoms but he felt completely fine. So, this patient of mine has never felt any discomfort or issues with 300 to 400 levels of sugar in routine without any medicines and leads as normal life like me and you.

Similarly, the IDEAL trial is one of its kind and the only trial that considers dialysis as a secondary treatment for kidney patients without any symptomatic discomfort. Generally with increased creatinine and decreased eGFR values, the kidney patients are prescribed to be on regular dialysis. However, according to IDEAL research it is not primarily necessary to prescribe dialysis even if the creatinine, uric acids, potassium and eGFR are undesirable, until the patient reports any symptomatic distress. Symptomatic discomforts like excessive fatigue, breathlessness, painfulness, dizziness, digestion issues or any minor/major disturbance of body and mind.

Even the ALLHAT trial sponsored by the government of US reported that, "High blood pressure with symptoms must only be considered for medical intervention." Reason being, it is not uncommon that individuals with blood pressure as high as 160/100 mmHg experience no symptomatic discomfort; rather feel completely comfortable as normal. Therefore, their body does not require blood pressure pills as they will create no difference but only lower down the readings (number value) on the recorder. That individual may remain healthy throughout his life with high readings; on the other hand, his condition may even deteriorate if unnecessarily medicated without any considerable symptoms. This is rather more dangerous.

This is to understand that to completely rely on modern technology based diagnosis is a grievous situation. Instead look for the warning signs that the body gives away, or symptomatic discomforts involved, as only these can be considered as the real indicating factors.

Metaphorically speaking, these days' Google maps are commonly used to locate and reach out to places conveniently. If you want to reach Taj Mahal, then you can take help of Google map to give you directions. Now suppose you have reached Taj Mahal but Google map directs you to travel another 2.5 kms to reach Taj Mahal, then whom will you trust - you, your eyes or senses as you can see the Taj Mahal in front of you or the Google map who wants you to travel another 2.5 kms and assume that place to be Taj Mahal. Obviously, you must believe in what you see, you must rely on your senses, not on technology; as too much dependency on technology leads to over-diagnosis.

Alas, the Medical industry does not want you to do so, rather directs instead deviates you from reality! Our medical industry has learnt to link disease with test reports. Once you have undesirable readings, then they search for disease to be linked and render you a patient to be dependent on medicines for lifelong.

To conclude, diagnosis is a trap laid by the modern medicine to convert a healthy individual into a permanent customer leading to the worst misery of the modern human, which often ends with the loss of life and wealth.

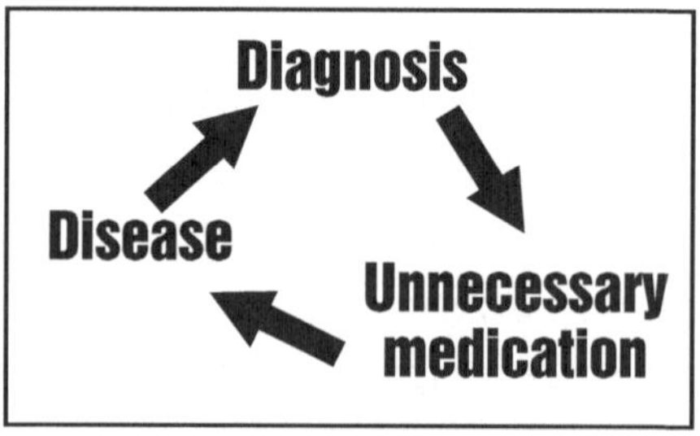

"You don't need medication,

You just need education"

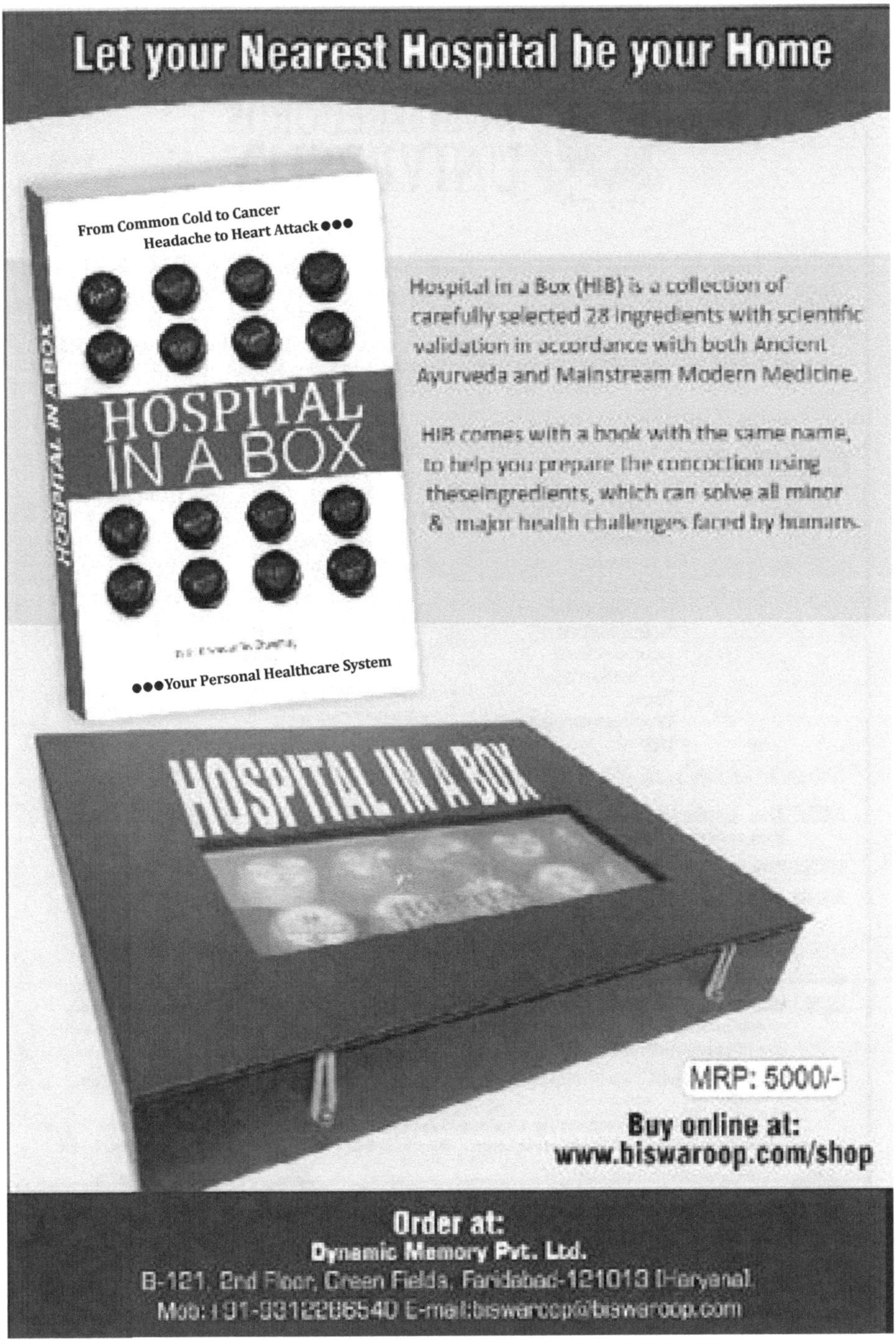
Let your Nearest Hospital be your Home
From Common Cold to Cancer
Headache to Heart Attack ●●●
HOSPITAL IN A BOX
HOSPITAL IN A BOX
●●●Your Personal Healthcare System
Hospital in a Box (HIB) is a collection of carefully selected 28 ingredients with scientific validation in accordance with both Ancient Ayurveda and Mainstream Modern Medicine.
HIB comes with a book with the same name, to help you prepare the concoction using theseingredients, which can solve all minor & major health challenges faced by humans.
HOSPITAL IN A BOX
MRP: 5000/-
Buy online at:
www.biswaroop.com/shop
Order at:
Dynamic Memory Pvt. Ltd.
B-121, 2nd Floor, Green Fields, Faridabad-121013 (Haryana).
Mob: +91-9312286540 E-mail:biswaroop@biswaroop.com

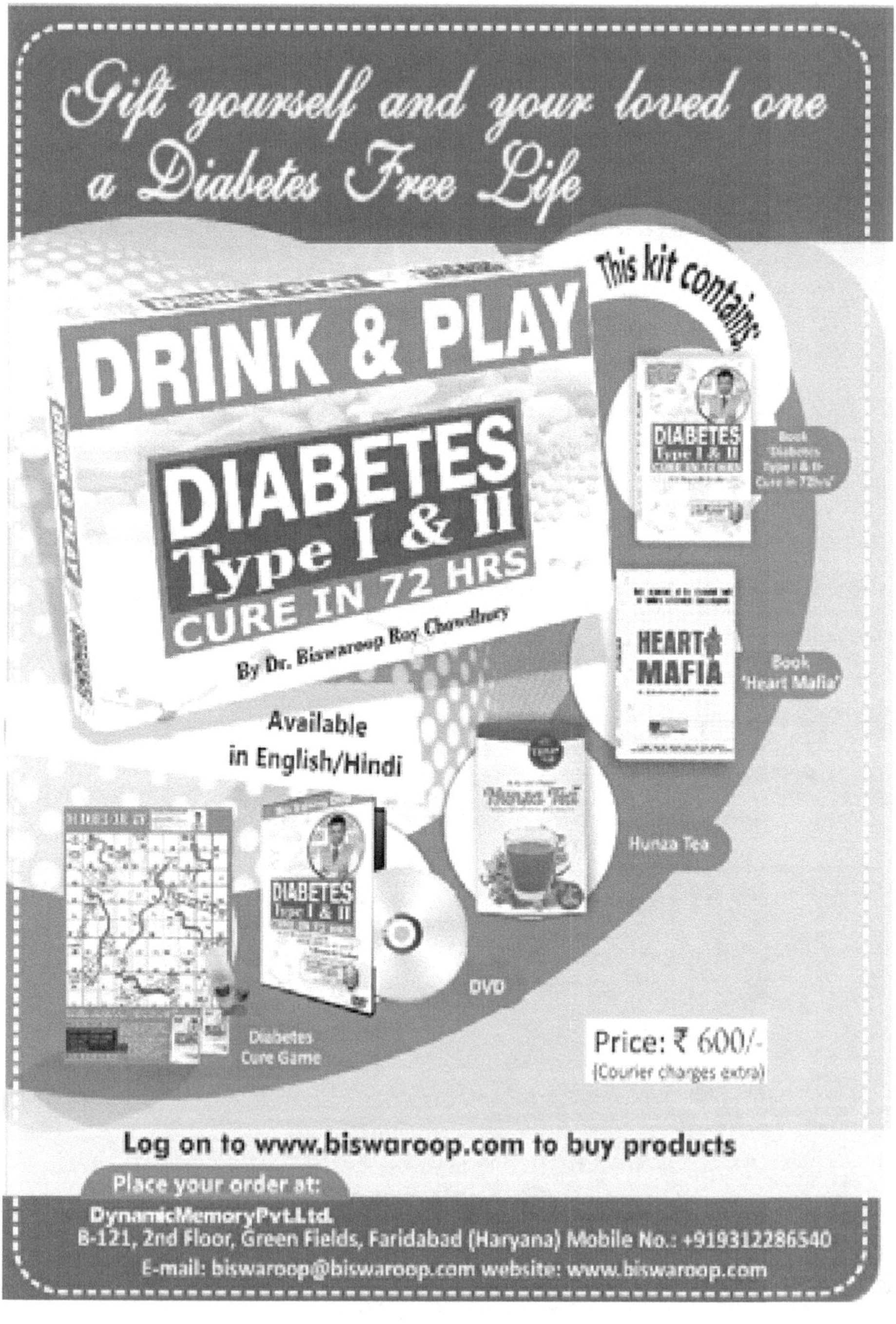
Gift yourself and your loved one a Diabetes Free Life
This kit contains
DRINK & PLAY
DIABETES Type I & II CURE IN 72 HRS
By Dr. Biswaroop Roy Chowdhury
Available in English/Hindi
HEART MAFIA
Book 'Heart Mafia'
Hunza Tea
DVD
Diabetes Cure Game
Price: ₹ 600/-
(Courier charges extra)
Log on to www.biswaroop.com to buy products
Place your order at:
DynamicMemoryPvt.Ltd.
B-121, 2nd Floor, Green Fields, Faridabad (Haryana) Mobile No.: +919312286540
E-mail: biswaroop@biswaroop.com website: www.biswaroop.com

Let every morning be the Hunza Morning

If you have decided to pick only one of my suggestions for the sake of your health. Then take this suggestion :

Stop consuming tea specially, morning tea. The early morning tea makes the inner lining of your intestinal wall acidic, as after night of fasting your stomach is empty and craving for food. An acidic stomach on a regular basis is the single biggest cause of all kind of inflammatory and lifestyle diseases including arthritis, diabetes etc.

How to stop craving of tea ⟶ Switch to Hunza Tea

Hunza Civilization: Hunza people are the Indians living at extreme northwest of India in Hindu Kush range. They are known to be one of the world's healthiest civilizations, often living up to the age of 110 years.

How to prepare Hunza Tea (serves four):

Ingredients:

- 12 Mint leaves(Pudina)
- 8 Basil Leaves(Tulsi)
- 4 Green cardamom (Elaichi)
- 2 gm Cinnamon (Dalchini)
- 20 gm Ginger (Adrak)
- 20 gm Jaggery (Gur)

Instructions:

- Take 4 cups of water in a tea pan
- Add all ingredients, simmer it for 10mins
- Add a dash of lemon juice and serve hot or cold